QUALITATIVE RESEARCH
PROPOSALS AND REPORTS

A GUIDE

OTHER WORKS BY PATRICIA L. MUNHALL

Nursing Research: A Qualitative Perspective (4th ed.)
The Emergence of Man into the 21st Century
The Emergence of the Family into the 21st Century
The Emergence of Women into the 21st Century
Nursing Research: A Qualitative Perspective (3rd ed.)
In Women's Experience (Volume I)
In Women's Experience (Volume II)
Revisioning Phenomenology: Nursing & Health Science Research

OTHER WORKS BY RON CHENAIL

Medical Discourse and Systemic Frames of Comprehension
Practicing Therapy: Exercises for Growing Therapists
The Talk of the Clinic: Explorations in the Analysis of Medical and Therapeutic Discourse
The Qualitative Report

QUALITATIVE RESEARCH PROPOSALS AND REPORTS: A GUIDE

THIRD EDITION

PATRICIA L. MUNHALL, ARNP, EdD, PsyA, FAAN
PROFESSOR AND PRESIDENT OF THE INTERNATIONAL
INSTITUTE OF HUMAN UNDERSTANDING
MIAMI, FL

RON CHENAIL, PhD
VICE PRESIDENT OF INSTITUTIONAL EFFECTIVENESS
AND PROFESSOR OF FAMILY THERAPY
NOVA SOUTHEASTERN UNIVERSITY
FORT LAUDERDALE, FL

JONES AND BARTLETT PUBLISHERS
Sudbury, Massachusetts
BOSTON   TORONTO   LONDON   SINGAPORE

World Headquarters
Jones and Bartlett Publishers
40 Tall Pine Drive
Sudbury, MA 01776
978-443-5000
info@jbpub.com
www.jbpub.com

Jones and Bartlett Publishers
Canada
6339 Ormindale Way
Mississauga, Ontario L5V 1J2
CANADA

Jones and Bartlett Publishers
International
Barb House, Barb Mews
London W6 7PA
UK

Jones and Bartlett's books and products are available through most bookstores and online booksellers. To contact Jones and Bartlett Publishers directly, call 800-832-0034, fax 978-443-8000, or visit our website, www.jbpub.com.

Substantial discounts on bulk quantities of Jones and Bartlett's publications are available to corporations, professional associations, and other qualified organizations. For details and specific discount information, contact the special sales department at Jones and Bartlett via the above contact information or send an email to specialsales@jbpub.com.

The authors, editor, and publisher have made every effort to provide accurate information. However, they are not responsible for errors, omissions, or for any outcomes related to the use of the contents of this book and take no responsibility for the use of the products described. Treatments and side effects described in this book may not be applicable to all patients; likewise, some patients may require a dose or experience a side effect that is not described herein. The reader should confer with his or her own physician regarding specific treatments and side effects. Drugs and medical devices are discussed that may have limited availability controlled by the Food and Drug Administration (FDA) for use only in a research study or clinical trial. The drug information presented has been derived from reference sources, recently published data, and pharmaceutical research data. Research, clinical practice, and government regulations often change the accepted standard in this field. When consideration is being given to use of any drug in the clinical setting, the healthcare provider or reader is responsible for determining FDA status of the drug, reading the package insert, reviewing prescribing information for the most up-to-date recommendations on dose, precautions, and contraindications, and determining the appropriate usage for the product. This is especially important in the case of drugs that are new or seldom used.

Library of Congress Cataloging-in-Publication Data
Munhall, Patricia L.
  Qualitative research proposals and reports : a guide / Patricia L. Munhall and Ronald J. Chenail.—3rd ed.
    p. ; cm.
  Includes bibliographical references and index.
  ISBN-13: 978-0-7637-5111-1 (alk. paper)
  ISBN-10: 0-7637-5111-1 (alk. paper)
  1. Nursing—Research—Methodology.   2. Qualitative research.   I. Chenail, Ronald J.   II. Title.
  [DNLM: 1. Nursing Research.   2. Qualitative Research.   3. Research Design.   4. Writing. WY 20.5
M966q 2008]
  RT81.5.M854 2008
  610.73072—dc22
                                                                                    2007023538
6048

Production Credits
Executive Editor: Kevin Sullivan
Aquisitions Editor: Emily Ekle
Associate Editor: Amy Sibley
Editorial Assistant: Patricia Donnelly
Production Director: Amy Rose
Associate Production Editor: Amanda Clerkin
Senior Marketing Manager: Katrina Gosek
Associate Marketing Manager: Rebecca Wasley
Composition: Auburn Associates, Inc.
Manufacturing and Inventory Control Supervisor: Amy Bacus
Cover Design: Timothy Dziewit
Cover Image Credit: ©Photos.com
Printing and Binding: Malloy, Inc.
Cover Printing: Malloy, Inc

Printed in the United States of America
11 10 09 08 07   10 9 8 7 6 5 4 3 2 1

To our students with gratitude, love, and respect. Each one, in his or her uniqueness, has taught us the meaning of the word gift.

Patricia L. Munhall
Ronald Chenail

Contents

Introduction

This is the third edition of the qualitative research proposal and report guide. Having used it in the classroom for several years and encouraging, and sometimes not needing to encourage students, we have asked for their suggestions before embarking on this edition. Along with their suggestions and those of colleagues, we have attempted to clarify some concepts, add a few more illustrations, update the references, and—new to this edition—include the numerous and valuable qualitative Web sites that provide critical information for the reader. We do not claim that these formats are like grant applications, though perhaps they should be for qualitative research. Rather, they are offered in the spirit of suggestion, to make what seems laborious or confusing somewhat more manageable. A long time ago, we became aware of the difficulty of using dissertation formats and research grant applications which patently seemed at odds with the flow and spirit of qualitative inquiry. We realized that in our research we listen, observe, read, become a part of something bigger than ourselves, become a part of the thing itself, dwell with thought, and interpret, while remaining wide awake and attentive to the appearance of the phenomenon of interest. How does one *fit* such processes into a proposal? How are those processes communicated into diagrams, or for that matter, structured *formats*?

However, we recall the need we once had for "the box"—the given format a professor might hand out at the beginning of a course and we have likened the box to a crib for a baby. Until the baby is safe to walk on her own, she needs the protection of a "box" to keep her from falling and hurting herself. Not unlike a map, we find safety and direction in steplike formulas, and so it is with this format guide that we provide some measure of guidance to students who are embarking on unfamiliar processes. Rather than perceiving the research as a steplike formula, we would encourage students to remain open and fluid to the flow of their own research and understand that on this "crib," the sides are down!

We have seen this guide changed by various instructors of the subject to fit more into their preconceptions and assumptions. Sometimes it is an improvement, and sometimes it is the introduction of incongruent philosophical underpinnings, and is not always congruent with qualitative research. We ask readers to be aware of this, and thus we stress the necessity of fully understanding the method you choose so that you can recognize congruency.

This little guide in no way takes the place of texts and courses on methods (this we emphasize throughout the book). Without the enriching influence of really knowing the method, of being inside and outside of it, using this book becomes a superficial exercise. We are confident that students know this, yet in the rush of everyday events, it is sometimes tempting to choose the path of least resistance. Please do not deprive yourself of the richness of this knowledge as written by those who haltingly and painstakingly helped evolve these methods. Every day, the interpretation of qualitative methods seems to grow, and the appreciation of their contribution to human science is not only acknowledged but also required for many projects and stands now as a legitimate, critical, comprehensive component of the human sciences. Qualitative methods embrace the situated context and contingencies of human experience and search for meaning in the lives of human beings. They offer opportunities to enrich the quality of life for people, affect public policy based on needs perceived by the population in question, and contribute to the design for evidence-based practice, which is evolved from the authentic voice and perception of those the human sciences exist to serve.

In many instances throughout this guide, we might sound like coaches, and it might be that we are. So we say with great encouragement and enthusiasm, reach out to individuals or groups, listen with all intensity taking in all that is there, and come back and tell us what you have found. Tell us how preconceived assumptions did not hold up, that a one-size-fits-all theory does not seem to hold up in the real world, and that people and groups are filled with secrets and surprises that we did not know before you did your research! Human understanding, theory development, and evidence-based interventions to improve the quality of life for all of us are waiting for you.

Patricia L. Munhall
Ron Chenail

About the Authors

Patricia L. Munhall, ARNP, EdD, PsyA, FAAN, serves as professor and president of the International Institute of Human Understanding. Formerly she was a professor at Hunter College, CUNY, and Columbia University. She is a noted authority on qualitative research methods, and the author of important works on qualitative research, phenomenology, and women's experiences. She is also a psychoanalyst practicing in Miami, Florida, United States.

Ron Chenail, PhD, is vice president for institutional effectiveness and professor of family therapy at Nova Southeastern University in Fort Lauderdale, Florida, and he is coeditor of *The Qualitative Report* and editor-in-chief of the *Journal of Marital and Family Therapy*. He is also a member of the editorial boards of *Counselling, Psychotherapy, and Health; Sistemas Familiares; Qualitative Research in Psychology;* and *Qualitative Social Work: Research and Practice,* and was a member of the founding editorial board of *Qualitative Inquiry.*

Doability

Our Aim

The influences that subtly affect our research enterprise bear critical examination because they have profound effects on outcomes. What we study and how we go about studying phenomena are often determined by the materials available to us. Whether these materials reflect quite different philosophical paradigms and systems of science or whether they reflect less tangible influences, it is important that we understand them (Crotty, 1998; National Research Council, 2002). Laudan (1977), in studying the less tangible, nonscientific influences on scientists, looked at the social forces influencing the community of scientists at a particular time. Currently, one such critical influence on our community of scientists involves existing proposal formats and guidelines that, for the most part, facilitate and frame quantitative or hypothesis testing designs of research. These proposals or formats are quite standard for dissertations, proposals, reports, research abstract submissions, grant applications, and publication of research. Because ac-

ceptance or rejection at any stage of research can be based on following the prescribed outline, the significance of such outlines or
materials must be addressed by the scientific community.

The purpose of this guide is to suggest a format or proposal that
would be appropriate for qualitative research designs in their broad
sense. At present, many qualitative researchers struggle to compress,
rearrange, and manipulate their *qualitative* research proposals into
existing materials too often designed specifically for *quantitative* research methods. Unfortunately, critical substance in these situations
often gives way to form. The processes of approval, acceptance, and
funding are philosophically and politically influenced by the formats available to us to frame our inquiries. Theory-building research,
however, needs distinctive formats to maintain the aim and integrity
of the particular approach and project.

Toward that aim, we suggest using flexible outlines for your qualitative research proposals as well as for your qualitative research reports and abstract outlines (see Tables 4-1, 9-1, and 12-1). Additionally, four figures (Figures 2-1, 4-1, 7-1, and 7-2) incorporate and
illuminate the possibilities of these outlines. We hope that they will
stimulate further thought and development as well.

None of these suggestions is presented as a vigorous method rule
or format. If there is one rule to follow in qualitative research, it
would be this: Let the data guide the way of inquiry (Chenail, 1995).
Guidelines, or lines of any kind, keep things back or out of sight.
Certainly such freedom can be difficult to deal with on one's first or
second qualitative research effort—thus, we offer these broad outlines to follow, as well as general indications on where to start and
where to go. However, during the study, if there is a pull in a certain
direction, then go with it—detours can sometimes lead to important
discoveries. However, as we will highlight in a later chapter of this
guide, never, ever forget the aim of your study! Another comment
about steps is that once we have completed a step we might have a
tendency to think that it *is* completed. This can lead to premature
closure, especially if we encounter new, additional data that is perti-
nent. So fluidity means to return to sections to amplify, as well
(Chenail, 1997).

In order to visualize these formats in actual studies, we have included three proposal formats and three completed research formats
in the appendices. Also, Table 4-2 (p. 18) is an example by one of us

(Munhall) of how this research format helped organize her proposal for a qualitative research project on understanding anger in women in therapy.

As with any suggested format, these formats are just that: *suggested*. Faculty, researchers and students may have differing ideas as to content and context based on what phenomenon is being studied. However, students and faculty who have been guided by this form have reported its helpfulness and the ways it enabled the qualitative process of inquiry to evolve. It is our hope that you will have a similar experience.

A caveat might be in order here. Oftentimes when there have been changes made to similar formats as these, the changes fall in two related categories. One is the attempt to still keep the formats as close to possible to the ones that are already established by the institution or granting agency. Related to that is the second category, and that is, in so doing, the changes seem to have origins in following the steps of the scientific method. An example of this is found in the beginning of the next chapter with a step for a theoretical framework or a review of the literature at the start of a qualitative study.

Our hope evolves that you shall be spared method errors and that you will be cognizant of the possibility that qualitative research formats might have erroneous steps. This calls for you to study the format that you are using, since it is very critical. To reiterate—which we will do a few times in this format book—this book does not prepare you for that kind of critique; only a solid understanding of qualitative research and its attendant processes can do that for you!

What Can Happen

Upon reviewing a student's qualitative dissertation proposal that had been written according to the quantitative research proposal outline for the student's institution, a doctoral committee found many compromises and inconsistencies. The first chapter of the proposal spelled out the required theoretical framework and a specific theory that the study would use. The proposal stated that the specific theory "will provide the theoretical perspective of the lived experience" of the phenomenon under study. The researcher then provided a full description of the preselected theoretical framework describing what is known about the subject of her study, and how she would be validating or testing the theory with her study (see Chapter 1 of this guide for warning of this type of deviation). The second chapter *of the same study*—on methodology—contained a quote from Omery (1983) saying that "to ensure that the phenomenon is being investigated as it truly appears or is experienced, the researcher must approach the phenomenon with *no pre-selected theoretical framework"* (p. 50, italics added). This, of course, placed the student researcher in a contradictory position. The material (i.e., the pro-posal format she had used) did not reflect her method: the substance and form were not philosophically or methodologically congruent.

While you are in the process of writing your proposal, know that the preceding ideas, in their general context, are still being discussed (i.e., whether any study can be truly atheoretical). In this regard, and for our purposes, a different perspective is suggested. As far as phi-losophy or theory is concerned, the *philosophy and theory of the method itself* gives direction to your study and should, therefore, be discussed congruently with or under that section (see Table 4-1, on page 17). You can also observe that there are *two sections not present* that are part of quantitative research studies and that can lead a researcher astray; one is the theoretical framework and the other the review of the literature.

For example, to do a phenomenological study, it is essential to un-derstand the philosophy of phenomenology and its philosophical underpinnings and to be able to view the world through the lens of phenomenological concepts (Munhall, 2007a,b; van Manen, 1990). You need to see through the lens of the method you are using, whether it is phenomenology (Munhall, 1994a, 2007a), narrative in-quiry (Clandinin, 2006), action research (Stringer, 2007), or another qualitative research method (Creswell, 2006). Some methodologists of grounded theory (Hutchison, 1993), for instance, speak about the theory of symbolic interactionism as the *undergirding theory of this method*. Sometimes there is confusion when doing a proposal, when a format asks for a theoretical or conceptual framework from which the study is derived. It is important to note the distinction here. Sym-bolic interactionism is the theory from which the *method* is derived, not the theory from which the *study* is derived. As was just men-tioned, in the formats suggested in this guide, you see the absence of theoretical or conceptual frameworks, keeping within the *atheoretical* philosophical underpinnings of qualitative research.

To reemphasize this critical distinction, if a format calls for a the-oretical framework before data collection, the format might be de-signed more for a quantitative study. If you are proposing to do a qualitative study, this is the time to discuss the philosophical and/or theoretical underpinnings of your qualitative method, as indicated specifically in Table 4-1, section III, letter b. It is important to understand that most likely there is a theory written about the phenomenon or subject you are about to study, but in qualitative research as you have learned, if you study the theory before collecting data, it could influence your perceptions and interpretations. You will research what is already in the literature in the later part of your data collection. This is the step in qualitative research where we say the literature review is postponed until after most data collection is completed for the same reasons, i.e., introducing bias and preconceived notions. In addition to reading the literature before hearing the authentic experiences of people or groups, the literature can be outdated, might not pertain to your group of individuals or culture, or might be acontextual and without the contingencies of your study. Figure 2-1 attempts to illustrate this unknowing openness perspective essential to qualitative research.

Thus we state in qualitative research that the research conducted is atheoretical but the method itself might not be. Returning to this distinction, our qualitative methods have very critical philosophical and theoretical substance or underpinnings and it is in section III of this book's research proposal format where you can espouse them and explain the foundation of the method to your readers (see Table 4-1, p. 17 and Table 4-2, p. 18).

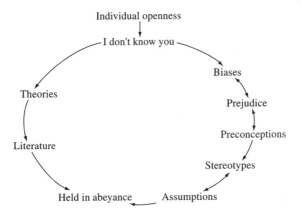

Figure 2-1 Unknowing Openness

Discussion of the method provides the researcher and the reader with a perspective that is necessary for understanding the study. Understanding the philosophy and assumptions of the method is essential to the critical thinking process of inquiry (Crotty, 1998). Individuals can easily follow steps, but to do so without understanding what the philosophical and theoretical foundation of those steps are can lead, metaphorically speaking, to a shallow, weak staircase in contrast to a thick, secure, safe staircase. You are substantially on better ground if you are confident about what is underneath you.

In the format we discuss throughout this book, section III is emphasized to help you as the researcher, and also to help your readers to understand the lens from which you are viewing your research aim, as well as your method. It will help you express more fully how philosophically and/or theoretically phenomenological, grounded theory, action research, narrative inquiry, or ethnographic methods, to name a few, perceive their individual research goals and procedures.

We believe the in-depth description of particular methods are essential to your own very understanding of what it is you are doing and also at this particular time in our research history in the human sciences, to also assist readers, many who have not been exposed to this level of articulation of qualitative methods. Contemporary criteria for best practices in qualitative research also call for a high degree of transparency in articulating the choices made in a study on the part of researchers as a sign of quality and integrity (see Anfara, Brown, & Mangione, 2002; Critical Appraisal Skills Programme, 2002; Russell & Gregory, 2003).

You might fully understand by now how our emphasis on critical study of method is essential before contemplating even a format! We want to assist you in that appreciation. It is the essence of your research.

The Need for Specific Guidelines

It has become apparent that specific guidelines for proposals for qualitative research methods are necessary in order to maintain the integrity of the research method. Broadly speaking, qualitative research is concerned with discovery (Mahrer & Boulet, 1999) and is, to the extent possible, atheoretical (as was emphasized in Chapter 2 of this guide). In contrast, *quantitative* research is more concerned with theory testing, validation, and confirmation. The latter starts with a deductive approach to hypothesis testing or theory testing (Chenail, 2000, 2005; Chenail & Maione, 1997; Munhall, 1994a, 1998, 2007a). Because the two approaches rest on different philosophical premises and methodological rules and processes, a proposal for a qualitative research design should differ substantively in syntax, logic, and process from that of a quantitative research design. In other words, *specific* guidelines for qualitative research proposals are essential and will facilitate qualitative researchers in articulating the aims and methods of qualitative studies.

As such, we present qualitative research proposal formats (Table 4-1, p. 17, and exemplar Table 4-2, p. 18) and qualitative research report formats (Table 9-1, p. 46, and exemplar Table 9-2, p. 49), as well as an outline for an abstract (Table 12-1, p. 64) for qualitative research. It is important to remember, as we have mentioned, the form is in the service of substance; whatever it may be, the form is quite secondary to the substance of the study. Still, in qualitative research proposals, in addition to being primarily attuned to substance, they must also provide:

1. Education about and description of the method, from its aim to its outcome.
2. Justification for using this method.
3. Translation of any unfamiliar language into words that will help the reader to understand the method better (Munhall, 1991, 2007a).

Provision for these processes fall within the following formats suggested within this book. These formats or guidelines have been used in major academic settings for over 15 years, for both masters' theses, doctoral dissertations, and other projects, such as grant applications for qualitative research. Some students and researchers have followed the guidelines precisely; others have used them as guides and made their own adjustments as their study progressed. However, as has already been discussed, caution must be used. Adjustments need to be philosophically congruent with the method. To reemphasize, the tendency to fall into the reasoning and steps of the scientific method is one of our major concerns. After lifetime careers in qualitative research, we still see students who have been ingrained with the scientific method way of thinking, struggling with a new way of thinking about and through research. Faculty members are often new to some of these methods, so students often find themselves in the unusual position of becoming the *expert* on a method. This is a wonderful opportunity to demonstrate what universities and granting agencies expound as one of their purposes—education and the search of truth—and no one ever said it had to be in a *one way direction*!

Faculty members are most eager to learn. After writing that sentence, we both want to add a caveat and in this age of *reality* everything, if you think a faculty member *does not fit that description*, please find yourself one who is excited about your project. In thinking further, no matter what, it is always an asset to find a faculty member who is or a granting agency that is truly committed to your research project. This is said from the perspective of this guidebook and as we said in the Introduction, your coaches!

Proposal for Qualitative Research Methods

Now is the time to critically study Table 4-1, Outline for Proposal for Qualitative Research Studies. As you can see, there are six sections to the proposal, the first four of which can probably serve as guides for your first four chapters. For example, if you go to the Table of Contents for Almquist-Copeland's, Becker's, and Lauterbach's proposals (see Appendices), you will see this format as it was followed and accepted. Table 4-1 provides a brief description of what can be incorporated into each chapter. Please read this with flexibility and with your own creativity flowing. Then go to Table 4-2 to review one of our own exemplars (p. 18). In this exemplar, you will see an actual proposal and amplification of what you might consider to discuss in these sections. Take note of section III, where a general discussion of a specific method goes from "what is it?" to the descriptions of the concepts and terms. All are essential for you and your readers to understand in an in-depth way (in this instance becoming phenomenological!). All qualitative methods need this kind of explanation.

You can also see that the chapters can be organized with subheadings as indicated by the letters in each section. This is illustrated in the study outline exemplars in Appendix B (p. 87), in which the studies themselves led to additional subheadings, demonstrating the richness of the studies and how the findings prompted new subheadings.

For now we will explore Table 4-1 and Table 4-2. As you study Table 4-1, you might wonder what exactly a, b, c, or d of any section means. Refer to Table 4-2 for examples. Some of the steps are what you expect in a research proposal, so they are standard. Others, such as section II, illustrate the intersubjective nature of a study by including you in the study, explaining how you became interested in the phenomenon or why you want to study a particular group. See Figure 4-1 for an illustration of the concept of intersubjectivity and its inherent shared perceptual space. When you study that figure, note that the more interaction between two people or between you and a group, the larger that shared perceptual space can become; therefore it is elastic.

Once again we acknowledge the repetitiveness of this *absolute need*, in order to understand this format book and in this example the various figures, you need to be grounded in qualitative research. If, while you are reading about a concept within this book and you are not sure of its meaning, for example, intersubjectivity (Schwandt, 2007), please return to your original books and textbooks (e.g., Creswell, 2006; Marshall & Rossman, 2006; Munhall, 2007a,b). We remember in the beginning of our own qualitative research endeavors, *the act of repeatedly returning* was essential to our own understanding.

Research proposals and reports inherently have some repetitive parts to them. For example, the aim is mentioned many times; however the aim is often repeated in another context for a different purpose. To us, the aim can never be thought of enough. We have each had students who lost sight of the aim of their study. We suggest you attach sticky notes in places you frequently look during the course of a day with the aim of your study announcing itself! Experience is filled with interesting diversions, and they can be fodder for your next studies. Remember this study *is all about your stated aim*!

Table 4-1   Outline for Proposal for Qualitative Research Studies

I—Introduction: Aim of the Study	a) Phenomenon of interest. b) Perceived justification for studying the phenomenon. c) Phenomenon discussed within specific context, e.g., a lived experience, a culture, a human response. d) Assumptions, biases, experiences, intuitions, and perceptions related to the belief that inquiry into the phenomenon is important. e) Qualitative research method chosen with justification of its potential. f) Relevance to discipline.
II—Evolution of the Study	a) Rationale. b) Historical context. c) Experiential context.
III—The Method of Inquiry: General	a) Introduction to a specific method. b) Rationale for choosing the method: philosophical and theoretical substantiation projected. c) Background of the method. d) Outcome of the method. e) Sources (individuals) whose methods will be followed. f) General steps or procedures of the method. g) Translation of concepts and terms.
IV—The Method of Inquiry: Applied	a) Aim. b) Sample. c) Setting. d) Gaining access. e) General steps. f) Human subject considerations: informed consent, entry, departure, confidentiality, secrets, process consent—if and when the situation should change. g) Strengths and limitations. h) Anticipated timetable. i) Actual feasibility of study—is access cost possible?
V—Appendices	a) Supporting documents. b) Consent forms. c) Communication.
VI—References	

Table 4-2 Abbreviated Exemplar of Proposal for Qualitative Research Studies

I—Introduction: Aim of the Study	a) Phenomenon	Understanding anger in women.
	b) Justification	Without understanding grounded in the perceptions of those who have experienced anger and are willing to describe the various outcomes, we do not have a basis for intervention for practice.
	c) Specific context	Women voluntarily coming into therapy with various problems—private practice.
	d) Assumptions	Previous experience led to assumptions.
	e) Method and justification	Phenomenology: to understand the meaning of experience and critique understanding.
	f) Relevance	Psychosomatic inferences of related illness to anger have social, health, and psychological implications.
II—Evolution of the Study	a) Rationale	Had begun to see instances of anger hidden within a physical, social, or emotional state of being.
	b) Historical context	Anger, as an emotional response, has a long history of attention, from healthcare providers to playwrights.
	c) Experiential context	I have felt angry, been the recipient of another's anger, and treated patients who had actual or related problems with anger.
III—The Method of Inquiry: General	a) Introduction	Phenomenology—what is it? Give a good philosophical description.
	b) Rationale	Method used to find meaning in experience.
	c) Background	Beginning history of phenomenology to present.
	d) Outcome	Understanding of meaning of experience.
	e) Source	Combination of van Manen and Munhall.

	f) General procedures
	g) Concepts and terms
IV—The Method of Inquiry: Applied	a) Aim
	b) Sample
	c) Setting
	d) Gaining access
	e) General steps
	f) Human subjects
	g) Strengths and limitations
	h) Timetable
	i) Feasibility
V—Appendices	a) Supporting documents
	b) Consent form
	c) Communication
VI—References	

f) Articulate the plan that will tentatively be used, knowing that the plan is flexible.

g) Terms such as *bracketing, intersubjectivity,* etc., need to be explained.

a) Understand the meaning of women's anger.

b) To include 10 patients, 10 women who are not patients, literature, films, diaries, biographies, art, anecdotes, personal journal.

c) Patients in a therapeutic setting, women in place of their choice, anecdotes from observation of day-to-day context.

d) Readily accessible. Patients and 10 women will be approached to participate.

e) Go through general steps as far as method, stress nonlinear nature.

f) Develop informed consent and obtain IRB approval.

g) Important topic with implications, perhaps too broad for one study.

h) Expected to last 2 to 3 years.

i) Very feasible: state why, along with foreseen reasons why not.

a) Letters and communications.

b) Consent forms.

c) Diagrams from method, etc.

Self-explanatory; however, include most on method and rationale for study.

Personal universes–Subjective views of reality

Intersubjectivity–Two views intersect

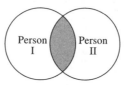

A shared perceptual field where subjectivities intersect

Figure 4-1   Shared Perceptual Space of Intersubjectivity

Composability

Aim of the Study

The aim of the study involves clearly articulating what it is you wish to accomplish. Is the aim to understand, describe, and interpret a particular phenomenon? If so, say it clearly and unambiguously. When stating an aim, it is preferable to err on the side of simplicity rather than complexity. In Table 4-2, p. 18, the aim is clearly stated to understand the meaning of repressed anger. A more detailed description of the aim is presented within the corresponding section of the proposal on anger, but the kernel is to understand repressed anger. Referring to Chapter 4 of this guide, this kernel would be the sticky note posted on your computer, refrigerator, wallet, doors, etc. As the researcher, you also need to communicate in the introduction of your proposal—or aim of the study section—the *perceived justification* for studying the phenomenon. Since a method for discovery is being used, the fundamental aim of the study will be to find out the answer to, "What is it like?" "What is this?" or "What's going on here?" Other questions can also be pursued, such as, "What is the meaning of this experience?" or questions probing cultural patterns or processes associated with certain social interactions. With action research, the inquiry can be guided with questions such as, "What is the nature of the problem facing the organization?" "What do we want to improve in our company?" or "What do we need to know about our institution before we can develop our plan?"

A specific problem statement would be premature at this point, as would be a research question with identified variables. This is because your research is designed to explore the phenomenon of interest without preconceived notions or hypotheses about presenting problems or predicted variables. This is critical to understand. Questions that include relationships between variables or comparisons between or among groups are usually not qualitatively oriented, however if you are doing a triangulated study (combining methods), such questions might be posed. It is strongly recommended that student researchers squelch the proverbial grandiose study that seems to be very gripping, as tempting as it may be. Instead, keep your study clear, crisp, and entirely focused. Triangulated studies seem only to complicate the matter. What you are studying should be reducible to four, five, or maybe six words. These are your sticky note words!

Additionally, the phenomenon should be discussed within the specific context in which you desire to study it. For example, "What is going on in a special type of nursing home?" "What is it like to feel healthy at a particular developmental phase, and why is this relevant to your field?" *Situate your study in the context in which it occurs.* Exploring rehabilitation settings in a qualitative inquiry, for example, would give us a description of the culture, patterns, and processes associated within that particular context. Problems can be discovered, areas where understanding and intervention are needed can become evident, and a theoretical base for hypothesis formation could be developed from the original field of study.

A *brief overview* of the qualitative method chosen by the researcher, along with its appropriate outcome, should be included in the introduction section of your proposal. As the researcher, your own experiences, intuitions, assumptions, and preconceptions can be included here as well, with reference to their further articulation in Table 4-1, sections II and III. In this regard, inclusion of such material in the introduction should be brief and elaborated on in the second chapter of your proposal. In the aim of the study section, you provide the information that is going to be elaborated upon in coming sections. This is the introduction to your study proposal. It is overarching, with details to follow.

The overall purpose of the introduction is to orient the researcher and reader to the phenomenon of inquiry and the broad design. It should convince the reader of *the importance of discovery and exploration* vis-à-vis a specific qualitative design. As the researcher, you also demonstrate in the proposal's introduction how the aim of the study has important implications and relevance for your research discipline. You demonstrate clearly the substance of the study. Table 4-1 suggests the items to be included. In your proposal, this will be Chapter I, which can be called the Introduction or the Aim of the Study, and if you are following this format, it would have six parts or six subheadings. You can elaborate what you say in the Introduction in Chapters II, III, and IV of your proposal.

This outline as proposed in Table 4-1 (p. 17) and Table 4-2 (p. 18) can be your outline for your own Chapter I. The appendices at the end of this book also demonstrate this format. We would like you *to understand the importance of this one particular chapter*. Sometimes like you, faculty members are overwhelmed with work, and readers might focus primarily on your introduction when reviewing your research proposal. Their first impression will be formulated while reading it. Polish this chapter so that it shines. Ask for critiques from your fellow students; ask if they understand what it is you are planning to do, ask for suggestions from others who can help you. There are also checklists available that you can use as a guide in your own self-evaluation (Mays & Pope, 2000), but we know it is often difficult to assess your own work. You know what you mean. The question is, have you communicated it well enough that others know what you mean as well? The introductory chapter is critical *and the clearer it is* as to your intent, the more you will have paved a road that you can congruently follow.

Evolution of the Study

In the evolution of the study, you place the study in the *context from which it has originated.* Readers of *quantitative* research proposals expect to understand, from a thorough literature review that supports the study, why the researcher is studying the phenomenon. In *qualitative* designs, the literature review is postponed in the interest of maintaining an open vision, one that is not theory-laden or biased, so that knowledge of the experience is, to the extent possible, without presuppositions and assumptions. Conceptual models and frameworks, if used this early in the study, might also selectively frame, or give direction to, the data. Like the literature review, they, too, can be brought in after data collection, when you want to establish how the findings of your study broaden, or are compatible or incompatible with a particular theory or conceptual model.

In a description of the evolution of the study, you again provide a rationale (Tables 4-1, 4-2, section II, a) for the study. Here you narrate the reason you have chosen this research aim, why it is significant to your discipline, and how it has the potential to increase knowledge for the betterment of your population. You should support this rationale within a *historical context*—that which you, the researcher, knows about historically—and an *experiential context*—that which is in your own experience. Here you should write of personal experience, which is often a starting point in exploratory studies. For example, you might write, "I came to realize that almost all the patients in the nursing home exhibited some signs of depression." Another example is given in Table 4-2, where a, b, and c of section II demonstrate the evolution of a study where one of us (Munhall) was researching the meaning of and implications of repressed anger. Often, this is where we see that the research interest originated somewhere in the researcher's practice or personal experience and has much to do with understanding a phenomenon that is of concern to that researcher within the context of his or her discipline.

The overall purpose of this chapter of the proposal is to describe the evolution of *your origin of interests,* to provide the reader with your rationale/reason for believing this study to be important, and to place the study in its historical and experiential context. Once again, when seeking a sponsor or committee members to be part of your research program, seek out those faculty members or granting agencies who share similar interests. The frosting on the cake would be to find a faculty member(s) not only with similar interests but also expertise in the qualitative method you have chosen. In a situation where this does not exist, for your own well-being and to assure quality guidance throughout this research experience, if you cannot find both qualities in one person, seek out a person with expertise in the content area and another person with expertise in the method you have chosen.

We express this concern along with our discussion of the evolution of your study, because we have seen the unfortunate fallout when students do not have the proper support. In order for your study to evolve successfully, choosing your committee members is not a task to take lightly or to finish quickly by asking whoever is available. Take time, investigate, and discuss your study with faculty members. Method expertise can be found in a faculty member outside your own department. This is not a step per se on the research format, but believe us, it is a crucial step not only for this research project but for

your own evolution as a researcher. Lastly, we suggest that you consult the relevant thesis or dissertation handbook under which your
study is being conducted in order to learn what criteria, if any, are in
place governing the selection of chairperson and committee members. Knowing these policies early in the process will save you time
and possible frustrations later in the development of your research
project.

The Method of Inquiry: General

The general method of inquiry is a critical component of the qualitative research proposal because of the need to educate readers who are not familiar with the method and to translate arcane terminology into a language accessible to the average reader. If, for instance, the researcher is going to use a phenomenological design, be it that of Merleau-Ponty (1956), Van Kaam (1969), Georgi (1970), Speigelberg (1976), van Manen (1990), or Munhall (1994a, 2007a), the processes need to be discussed in the clearest terms. This is where both *education* and *translation* come into play. For example, phenomenological terminology is not always understood by and is often not within the experience of many faculty members, researchers, or readers of research.

Words or expressions such as "the study of essences," "a caring attunement," "embodiment," "primacy of perception," and "reviewing contacts with original experience" need to be translated into simpler terms. Statements such as "phenomenology begins in silence" and "we become the question" are not always comprehensible to the reader. Also, you, as the researcher, can actually profit from a thorough translation, because it often requires you to confront the concepts to be explained with your own experience, thereby resulting in a deepened understanding both of these concepts and your experience. We use phenomenology in this discussion deliberately because many of the concepts found in phenomenological philosophy will also be undergirding other qualitative research methods. If you chose a grounded theory method or action research, you will have specific concepts and processes to explain and describe.

Sometimes diagrams provide help in understanding the general description of the inquiry. Such diagrams can then be utilized again in the following section on methods *applied*. Three diagrams are included here that we believe are compatible with van Manen's (1990) interpretations of phenomenology. For example, Figure 7-1 can communicate to the reader where your data might come from in a phenomenological study. In Figure 7-2, you should specifically spell out in the particulars of the study the phrases or words as they apply to the specific method you are using. Figure 7-3 should help you with the space-time, embodiment, and the relational part of the particular method you are using (Munhall, 1994a, 2007b). The interconnectedness of time, body, space, and relationships all contribute to making sense out of data and need to be acknowledged as simultaneous interactions inherent in your data. Yes, this might be another teaching moment when we remind you to *return* to your literary resources to fully understand, for example, the importance of the life worlds in all qualitative research and their embedded interconnectedness and implicate order (Bohm, 1985; Munhall, 2007b).

Pragmatically speaking, these guidelines can keep you oriented and organized. Other methods can generate similar diagrams. Remember, though, that whatever method and language you use to describe, it must be clear. This methodological presentation might be made in Chapter III of your proposal, so look at Table 4-1, III (p. 17) and make sure you include in this chapter, a) the introduction to your method, b) the rationale for choosing the method, c) the background of the method, d) the outcome of the method, e) sources of the method you will be following, f) general steps or procedures of the method, and g) the translation of the concepts and terms, as we discussed.

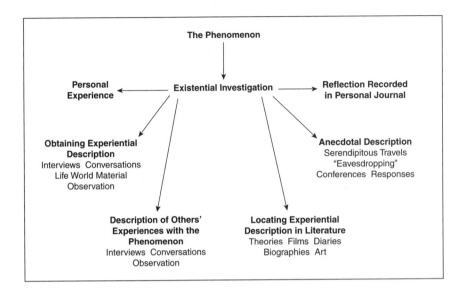

Figure 7-1   The Phenomenon-Existential Investigation

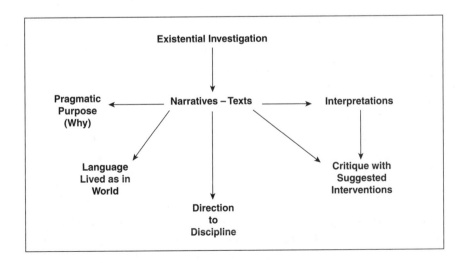

Figure 7-2   Existential Investigation-Narrative-Texts

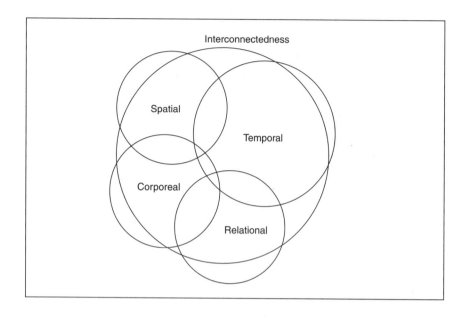

Figure 7-3   Four Existential Life Worlds

In grounded theory, *basic social processes, core variables* and *theoretical codes* are phrases that need translation. When describing the method, it is in your best interest to translate the conceptual language of that method into familiar, understandable terms. As is the case with the various phenomenological approaches to inquiry, when you are using grounded theory, you must also take care to consistently acknowledge the variant of grounded theory methodology being employed in the study (e.g., Glaserian or Straussian; Heath & Cowley, 2004).

The general method of inquiry section of your proposal is primarily concerned with the process of the *specific qualitative method itself,* whereas the next section is devoted to applying the method to your study. In years to come, this section might not be necessary; at the present time, however, this overview of methods is critical to the understanding by faculty members, grant reviewers, and students of how the researcher is going to use a given method, and *how that method works.* You thus introduce in a readily readable language the specific method and give the rationale for choosing the method and the philosophical underpinnings. The background of the method, as well as the outcome and importance of this type of method, need to be emphasized; that is, you must emphasize what the method will produce for your discipline, and why it is important.

If, for instance, the identification of basic social processes within a setting helps create enhanced interventions, it should be highlighted. If a phenomenological baseline is critical to theory development, it needs to be underscored. In action research projects, it would be important to note what action-reflection cycle will be governing your project (e.g., planning, acting, observing, or reflecting; McNiff & Whitehead, 2002). An overview of the process, including a brief description of what each step entails, should comprise this chapter of your proposal in a *generic* form; the following chapter of your proposal will be the *application* of this method as planned for your specific study, as stated earlier.

Do this chapter well, not only from the perspective of *writing* the chapter but also from the perspective of *learning* your method thoroughly in a way you understand and about which you can communicate clearly. You must know the inside and outside of this method, as well as the permeable circumference.

The Method of Inquiry: Applied

In the applied method of inquiry section of your proposal, it would be helpful for you to repeat *the aim of the study,* and then to show *how* the actual application of the chosen method will *accomplish the aim.* You then go through the procedure as discussed in Chapter 7 of this guide, but now with the details of the specific study. In grounded theory, for example, the researcher describes how the processes of memo writing, sorting, saturation, literature review, and conceptualization are to be carried out within the specific parameters of his or her particular study (Strauss & Corbin, 1998).

With most *quantitative* methods, the sample needs to be selected according to preestablished guidelines. However, in *qualitative* studies, *sample* size might not be as important as it is for quantitative studies for different reasons. When interviewing individuals about a particular phenomenon, one might, for instance, continue the interview process with as many individuals as it takes until no new information or new interpretations by the research participants becomes available. When repetition or redundancy appears in the data, gathered either from a single individual or a group, the saturation point might have been reached, and it appears that there is no new information to be obtained at that time. If saturation occurs in your study, discuss this event and provide your rationale for believing that saturation has occurred. Sometimes in qualitative research, such as narrative inquiry, the researcher might decide the number of narratives that he or she wishes to have in the study. As long as a good rationale is given, that is acceptable. A study can consist of a single case study! In action research, you would discuss how sampling would be managed within each of the parts of a particular cycle (e.g., planning or observing). For example, you most likely would need to reach a degree of saturation in any one of the cycle parts before you reach a level of confidence, suggesting it is time for you to progress to the next step in the cycle (McNiff & Whitehead, 2002).

In the applied method of inquiry section, when discussing the sample, you must communicate the characteristics of, as well as the *rationale* for the selection process. Suggestions for selecting participants or sites to be used in qualitative research studies can be found by *returning* to texts that deal with particular methods.

The *setting* and how you are going to gain access must be described. The phenomenon of study guides the selection of both the setting and the sample. The departure from a quantitative format consists of describing, in a systematic way, how you will go about obtaining experiential descriptions from subjects.

In keeping with the generated expectations of readers and reviewers, this section of your proposal should also include the details—format and procedure—of the planned interviews, the planned observations and techniques, the way data will be stored, and the particulars of *reliability* and *validity* of the method used. When contemplating qualitative research, you need to explain, in clear terms, how you address the concepts of reliability and validity. For example, most qualitative reviewers have substituted different criteria for evaluation than the formalized definitions of reliability and validity that are used for quantitative research (Drisko, 1997). A good source text on the specific method of concern can provide this information. However, this information must be translated into language that is perfectly accessible and accurate to the study. In *Reliability and Valid-*

ity in Qualitative Research, for example, Kirk and Miller (1986) explain and distinguish among three kinds of reliability: quixotic, diachronic, and synchronic (see also Sandelowski, 1986). Mackey (2007) gives an overview of evaluation of qualitative research, including criteria from different disciplines and for different methods. Clive Seale's 1999 work, *The Quality of Qualitative Research,* is another good work to consult when questions of reliability, validity, trustworthiness, and rigor arise. As a qualitative researcher, you indeed have a challenging task, not only in presenting a proposal, but also in translating and teaching a method.

Human subject considerations and means of human subject protection should be included in this section of your proposal as well. In addition to traditional concerns, you need to address the handling of entry, departure, secrets, interviews, observations, and information from the perspective of protecting individual rights. It is also advisable to describe process consent, whereby reviewing and/or renegotiating any informed consent made with subjects is done from the perspective of the dynamic quality of field work or sequential interviewing (Munhall, 1988, 2007a). We also suggest you consult with your governing institutional review board (IRB) representative and familiarize yourself with the policies and procedures involved with securing approval to conduct your study with human subjects. Depending on the design being proposed for the study, some IRBs have raised significant issues resulting in substantial delays and multiple revisions, so it would be prudent to investigate this area of oversight and develop appropriate strategies in order to best manage this review process (Lincoln & Tierney, 2004).

Plans for the dissemination of findings should also be included. In qualitative studies and as part of the validity process, findings are often discussed with the participants to ascertain accuracy in reporting. Additionally, you will want to communicate the findings of the dissertation or a research report to a granting agency to professional or community audiences, as well as in journals or other kinds of literature. Participants to be included in your study should be consulted and must agree in writing as a condition of human subject protection. This is part of informed consent. It is critical in most instances that participants' identities are never revealed, in other words *the findings are not confidential, but the participants are anonymous.* We urge you to take the time to discuss this with your participants or groups, so that there will not be a misunderstanding later. Your chairperson or IRB representative can also assist you with determining the best ways to manage this process.

You must also include the *strengths and limitations* of your study by reiterating the study's relevance to your field of study and the importance of the particular method used. For emphasis, why this particular research interest lends itself to a qualitative study can be restated in this section as a particular strength. While we cannot ignore limitations, the usual references to sample size, generalizability, or probability should not be listed as limitations *since they do not hold the same meaning for qualitative research methods* as they do for quantitative research methods. It is also unnecessary to state that the researcher has little familiarity with the method that imposes a limitation. That has little to do with the method chosen, whether qualitative or quantitative. Even if this is the first study you have done, who is to say that it might not be the best! Limitations are easier to identify once the study has been completed, but you might mention potential limitations beforehand. For example, even though generalizability is not something qualitative researchers are concerned about, one could say a limitation is that the findings only pertain to a certain set of individuals. In the anger study in Table 4-2, this would be women in therapy, which comprised half of the sample (in phenomenological research, though, there is additional data that is used . . . the plot thickens, and it is time again to *return* to your texts).

Include in this chapter of your proposal your anticipated timetable and the actual feasibility of your study; that is, state that it is possible! Discuss why you are making such claims.

APPENDICES

For the most part the appendices section is similar to those of quantitative research methods, and it includes communication, consent forms, proof of human subjects' approval, and other supporting documents.

REFERENCES

References should be listed according to the style manual designated by your institution.

BRAVO

If you have followed all of the steps in this guide to this point, your proposal is done!

Completability
and Expectability

Reporting Qualitative Research Studies

When the qualitative study is completed, you are ready to write the findings of the inquiry. The proposal, initially written in the *future tense* as a plan, is written in the *past tense* as a report of activities that have transpired and are included in the whole research report or dissertation. In section V and section VI of your report (see Tables 9-1 and 9-2), you *return to the present tense*, which will sometimes speak to the future! The first four sections (see Table 9-1) can remain almost as they were in your proposal, shortening or lengthening the content depending on the projected audience. Table 9-2 provides an example.

Table 9-1 illustrates that the initial sections of your report or dissertation—Chapters I through IV—are mainly consistent with your proposal, except for changes or alterations that needed to take place. We now turn our attention to sections V and VI of Table 9-1, which addresses the results, implications of, and reflections on your completed study. Although not illustrated here, an additional chapter can

Table 9-1   Outline for Reporting Qualitative Research Studies

I—Aim of the Study	a) Same as the proposal but with more breadth. b) Include new outline of remaining report. Transitional paragraph as explained on p. 57.
II—Evolution of the Study	a) Same as proposal. b) More breadth and depth.
III—The Method of Inquiry: General	a) Same as the proposal but more specific.
IV—The Method of Inquiry: Applied	a) As it happened.

V—Findings of the Inquiry	a) Findings are discussed according to the method. Example: In grounded theory method, the aim is generation of theoretical constructs. In this section, then, you would have findings from the process of:
	  • memo writing
	  • theoretical sampling
	  • sorting
	  • saturation
	  • the review of literature
	  • developing the theory
	b) With the ethnographic method, the findings may be reported in a smooth, flowing description narrative. The aim of the narrative is to portray the full context, to the extent possible, which was discovered by exploring pieces of reality and/or experience. Review of other sources, such as literature, art, and films is a plus.
	c) With phenomenology guiding the method, the findings will be reported differently. An example might include:

- a description of experiential themes
- a description of the essences of experience
- a description of relationships among essences
- a review of other sources (literature, art, films)

d) With action research, the findings would be reported in terms of the goals and outcomes for each phase in the cycle of inquiry. An example might include:

- a description of the problem or issue
- a description of the proposed intervention and implementation plan
- a report of findings from the assessment of intervention implementation
- articulation of the next steps in the resolution of the problem or issue and the future status of the intervention

VI—Reflections on the Findings	a) Meanings and understandings.
1. With preconceptions and ideas as discussed in the introduction.	b) Implications of the study (for whom).
	c) Relevance of the study (for whom)
2. With existing literature and practice in the area of study.	Integrate the following:
	d) Significance and substance.
	e) Importance to discipline.
3. With the utilization of the method.	f) Critique of findings with suggestions for change and future inquiry.

REPORTING QUALITATIVE RESEARCH STUDIES

Table 9-1 *(continued)*

VII—Appendices	Dissertation proposals and reports would include all necessary appendices, e.g., consent letters, tables, etc.

VIII—References

Source: Both the exemplars for the tables in this chapter have been taken from Munhall, P. (1994) *The Transformation of Anger into Pathology.* In P. Munhall (Ed.). In *Women's Experience,* New York: National League for Nursing Press, New York, 1994 (available from Jones and Bartlett, Sudbury, Mass.) and also Munhall, P. (1993) *Women's anger and its meanings: A phenomenological perspective.* Health Care Women Int.*14*(6):481–91.

Table 9-2   Abbreviated Exemplar of Outline for Reporting Qualitative Research Studies (Continuing With Anger Proposal)

I—Aim of the Study	This section of the report contains more breadth and description about the aim and the need to understand the meaning of the experience of anger. Remember this is in the past tense and you have completed your study so you can contribute more to all sections. In a phenomenological study on anger, the study is written in the first person and contains much of my own experiential and observational experiences.
II—Evolution of the Study	More breadth and discussion as to the evolution of the study; add more to the rationale, now that you know more about the importance of the study; add to the historical context if additional material has come to light; and experientially, it may be self-disclosing (this is a personal decision). See note above on experiential material.
III—The Method of Inquiry: General	This section will contain any changes you have made from your original description of the method of inquiry: general.
IV—The Method of Inquiry: Applied	May be the same or have become enlarged. For example, if you believe that the material of phenomenology leads you to different sources of material, you will find that your applied section has greatly expanded with your own creativity and imagination. For example, in the study of anger, Experiential and existential data included films, social context, societal norms, paradoxes, patient stories, transformative forms of anger as pathology, novels, and scientific literature, to name a few.
V—Findings of the Inquiry	[In this exemplar we will discuss only the phenomenology part, i.e., section c).] The findings of the inquiry led more to a narrative than a listing of themes or essences, which I have come to believe are not as helpful as narrating the meaning of experience (see Munhall 1993, 1994b). Examples from Munhall, 2007b) include:

Table 9-2 *(continued)*

- a contextual analysis of a film
- a social-historical analysis on the repression of anger
- the paradox of anger
- transformation of anger into physiological disorders; this warranted a longer description in narrative
- what is acceptable treatment today and why that treatment, within the context of this study, is inappropriate
- transformation into psychological disorders
- transformation into social problems
- repression, silence, concealment

The findings are unique to each qualitative study.*

VI—Reflections on the Findings:		
1. With preconceptions and ideas as discussed in the introduction.	a) Meaning	a) Meaning of anger is explicated and dramatically influential in women's lives.
	b) Implications	b) Implications have meaning, I believe, for individuals who are suffering and/or for healthcare professionals. For example, placing women on diets, when the underlying dynamic is anger.
2. With existing literature and practice in the area of study.	c) Relevance	c) Relevance of the study is very broad and was described as such as the study evolved; the study was apparently not to be completed but to be ongoing.

Table 9-2 *(continued)*

3. With the utiliza-tion of the method.	d) Significance	d) Repression and transformation of anger were integrated into the study.
	e) Importance to nursing	e) Understanding concealed the dynamic hiding behind the presenting condition.
	f) Critique	f) Understanding of the negative consequences leads to suggestions to provide women with healthy ways to discharge anger. Further inquiry is encouraged to expand knowledge of the transformation of anger into such powerful negative forces.

VII—Appendices

VIII—References

*This table accentuates in the Table 12-2 other ways of articulating the findings of this study.

Source: Both the exemplars for the tables have been taken from Munhall, P. (1994). *The Transformation of Anger into Pathology.* In P. Munhall (Ed.), In *Women's Experience.* New York: National League for Nursing Press (available from Jones and Bartlett, Sudbury, MA) and also Munhall, P. (1993) *Women's anger and its meanings: a phenomenological perspective.* Health Care Women Int. *14*(6):481–91.

involve an activity in which some researchers might wish to engage: a narrative detailing the entire research project itself. Such a chapter would be a 12–15 page complete summarization of your study.

We mention this because there is value in writing a chapter that actually *could become one of your research publications*. Not many institutions require this, but we urge you to keep this in mind. Your research is fresh, you will be receiving critiques, and you will be in a prime position to move to publication (see Chamberlain, 1999; Germano, 2005; Luey, 2004; for more advice on publishing from your dissertation). We are only human; once the dissertation is complete, often we wait too long to publish our studies. This is unfortunate both for you and your discipline, so we urge you to give some thought to *writing this extra chapter* or separate manuscript while you are still in the research process.

To visualize these sections, you should now look at the Tables of Contents used by Becker, Almquist-Copeland, and Lauterbach for their final doctoral dissertation studies (see Appendix B). You can see how following the outline described in this book helped the logic and organization of these students' very fine studies. Chapter IV (or section IV, Table 9-1) in the proposal, *Method of Inquiry: Applied*, while remaining consistent (if all goes well), could change in the report to accurately and particularly reflect how the method was actually carried out. When planning research we cannot foresee what we might have to revise. Also after studying Table 9-1, note how Table 9-2 also reflects the application of the format using the ongoing example found in the anger study.

In writing Chapter IV of your report, describe *specifically* how the method was used in accomplishing the aim of the study. If you utilized the grounded theory method, then the details of data gathering need to be described clearly: how you coded the field notes; used memos; did theoretical sampling, sorting, and saturation; reviewed the literature; and so forth (Strauss & Corbin, 1998). This section can be subdivided to include the literature review after the observations and interviews of data collection are completed. Oftentimes with qualitative research methods, the literature review is *considered part of the data collection* (Ryan & Bernard, 2003). The researcher may, for instance, present the interviews, the participants' observation activities, and then a literature review, in that order. Other sources of data to be collected about any given phenomenon through a qualitative lens might include art, films, documentaries, poetry, and other aesthetic forms that express the lived experience and/or culture of concern. This is illustrated in Table 9-2, section IV. This can be discussed in both chapters III and IV of your report (or sections III and IV, Table 9-1), illustrating repetition with a different rationale.

You will find yourself discussing the sample, setting, human subject considerations, and evaluation criteria as you compare what you wrote in your proposal to the reality of what occurred and the reasons for changes. What happens in the field usually cannot be predicted when writing your proposal. This chapter then is your method of inquiry. Initially, you described it generically in your proposal, but in your study report you fully discuss what actually occurred in your utilization of the qualitative method.

Keep in mind that section IV or what might be Chapter IV of your study report is a discussion on your use of the method and changes in the method, but not actual content of the findings. A good book leads up to an exciting finish, where the reader finds out how the story ends. Likewise, your report's exciting finish is the findings!

Findings of the Inquiry

Section V of Table 9-1 (p. 46) varies in narrative style so as to portray to the fullest extent possible the experience and observations that you have discovered, explored, and interpreted. *Depending on the method,* this is where style varies in that some qualitative findings lend themselves to be thematically analyzed, perhaps developed into tentative theoretical suppositions, synthesized into a descriptive narrative of a specific culture, or findings of how a group has been empowered by a change in the environment. Although diagrams could be used to enhance the narrative (Harry, Sturges, & Klingner, 2005), for the most part this section is in prose. It may be phenomenological writing, writing of a grounded theory, or writing a narrative about a specific culture or subculture. As the writer, through words, you articulate findings, and while they are your findings, they should *faithfully reflect the narrative and the portrait of the subjects.*

After doing all the activities required in data collection, and with such great immersion in the phenomenon, just what did you find out? What was in your journal (if you kept one), what did people say, what did people experience, what did you find in literature or in the media? Did you find photographs, poems, or other forms of art? In this section, you should use the words of your participants (their stories), write about films, or use literary quotes and whatever other material that spoke to you about the essence of your study. Everything you said you were going to do in your study proposal is discussed in this chapter of the study report by describing what you found. These findings are written according to the method you have chosen. Specific suggestions for writing the findings for your particular method are found in textbooks specific to that method (e.g., Crang & Cook, 2007, for ethnographies; Goulding, 2002, for grounded theory; Herr & Anderson, 2005, for action research; Munhall, 2007a,b, for variety of methods, including phenomenology).

Qualitative methods are continually evolving; during the last decade, methods have been further delineated so that there are many more methods available for specific purposes (e.g., authoethnography, Ellis, 2004; synergic inquiry, Tang & Joiner, 2006; and rapid assessment process, Beebe, 2001). Each of these methods has a particular way of reporting the findings, and most important, each method is searching for different kinds of findings, keeping within the scientific and philosophical underpinnings of qualitative research.

We want to emphasize once again to use the appropriate texts as to the method you are using from the beginning to the end, but in reporting the findings it is of critical importance. If you are reporting an ethnographic study, you should discuss ethnographic findings, not phenomenological findings. However, sometimes you do find other qualitative findings outside of your specific method! You can include them, but identify them appropriately. As we have said elsewhere; do not go too far astray from the aim of your study. For example, often in ethnographic studies one does find phenomenological findings. In a case such as this, phenomenological findings can be written as a separate manuscript or used as a foundation for your next research project. *Remember once again the aim of your study.* Sometimes in the findings section of a report, there is a tendency to wander into different areas (see Chenail, 1997). Call attention to these areas as areas for future study, but without equivocation concentrate on fulfilling the aim of your study.

The authors have both sat on dissertation hearings, to hear readers ask our poor researcher, "what does this have to do *with your study?*" This is a good question, and we suggest you ask it of yourself as you are writing the findings of your study. As you keep this in the forefront of your reporting of the findings, you reconstruct the inquiry within the context in which it occurred, the variations, the similarities, and the surprises. Summarize this section with a paragraph of the findings and a lead in sentence to Chapter VI of your report, Reflections on the Findings.

In your study report, always end each chapter with a summary of that chapter and a sentence leading into the next chapter. Always start a chapter with an introductory paragraph of what that chapter is going to be about. It seems elementary, dear Watson; yet we tend sometimes to forget our English teacher in the 10th grade, and that is a big mistake! He or she taught us the importance of transitional sentences. In our theme of *returning,* you might need to return to a good writing manual.

Reflections on the Findings

In following section VI of Table 9-1 (p. 46), discuss the *meaning* of your findings. What are the *understandings* gleaned from the findings, and what are the possible implications? This section of your report should also bring the inquiry together as a whole, including a comparison and discussion of the findings with the preconceptions and ideas as discussed in the first section of the proposal. Attention should be called to the context of the study as you reflect on and interpret the findings. Any information that appears in the literature on the phenomenon, culture, basic social processes, or the intervention, for example, of action research also needs to be discussed. Reflections on the method and its outcome should enter this discussion along with suggestions for future inquiries.

This should be a deeply reflected-upon chapter, where the findings have been critically thought about and discussed with others for additional insights or possibilities. The authors have found the most potential for additional insights is to discuss our findings, unless it would be inappropriate, with our participants or groups. Whose lives are we writing about? Surely our participants can see if we are getting it right. Thus we discuss meanings and understandings we gleaned with our participants. We talk about possible implications as well *with* our participants and also with our colleagues. Too often research becomes an isolated activity and we do not use those around us to our best advantage. In the reflections of the findings section of your report, discuss those to whom the study is relevant, to those we serve or the discipline itself, to public policy and/or the general public. What is the significance of this study to these groups?

Very critical to qualitative studies (and also quantitative, though that is not what we are discussing!) is the process of critique (Crotty, 1998; Munhall, 2007a,b). In this chapter on the reflections of the findings, you must critique your findings and interpretations and recommend suggestions and strategies to improve your human science field. It is here where you should include recommendations based on your findings for political, social, healthcare, family, and other social systems. In the next chapter of this guide, we will discuss how essential it is to communicate the critique to the individuals who might foster change or continued investigation, if the case may be. It is a shame that many studies reveal findings that are very troublesome, counterproductive to various practices, or that report dehumanizing conditions, and yet never reach the right audience. Please take seriously your ethical responsibility, the very foundation for our research, to improve the quality of life of those we serve. There has been discussion that if researchers reveal negative findings, it will be difficult for other researchers to gain access to the field. We find these discussions appalling. We have a moral imperative to bring to light our findings, both the good and the bad. Please discuss this with your faculty advisor, for guidance and suggestions. Of course, not every study results in such a dilemma.

At the very end of your study the most important evaluation question might be, "so what?" Believe us, this question comes up! With your study it should be evident, so that the question does not even come to mind. Start with an *important* aim and end with a meaningful critique that focuses on a positive change producing positive outcomes.

An important human consideration is to be faithful and thoughtful with respect to the language of your study participants and to their customs, beliefs and values. These considerations should be close to the world from which they originated. If possible, the poetry of the individuals' descriptions should be captured. Your attentiveness to their feeling states should be reflected in your writing. In other words, qualitative writing should reflect the highest degree of respect, sensitivity, and empathy.

Most qualitative researchers who have studied human phenomena or experience in this manner are quite moved and touched by their experiences during the research process. Some are even astonished. When these researchers begin to write, one of their greatest challenges is to communicate the simple, the complex, the joy or sadness, and perhaps pain to the reader (Gilbert, 2000). When you write your report, allow your readers to be as moved, touched, or astonished as you were. Remember, your ultimate goal is to help others understand some thing as you have. When reading over the last two chapters of your report, be attentive to that goal, and ensure that you reach it. Your ultimate questions are: Have I clearly and articulately fulfilled the aim of the study as stated at the beginning? Have I conveyed the "whatness of it all" and "the wholeness of it all," and have I made it understandable? Additionally, have I, through my critique, suggested ways that encourage the positive findings, and also strongly suggested ways to alleviate pain and suffering and potential ways to solve discovered problems? Have I completed a study that will contribute to the quality of life of living beings? You do not have to solve the problems per se; what is critical in your research is that you have found essential areas that need further research.

Please commit to disseminating your suggestions concerning that last question, to the widest audience possible. "Make your study count!" say your coaches!

APPENDICES

Include in your appendices all necessary information not discussed in the body of the work, including copyright information, informed consent forms, human subject approval, or institutional review board letters and any other relevant material.

REFERENCES

Using your institution's required writing manual, thoroughly comb your entire research report, making sure all needed material is present, that all material is accurately quoted and proper recognition is given to its author, and that all material needing references is so referenced accurately.

ENCORE!

As we closed in the proposal discussion, we will close the report discussion with a respectful, *bravo!* Now we add, *encore!*

Abstract

To be helpful to researchers, planners of research conferences often provide a format for submitting research abstracts. This can be enormously helpful, to the extent that the abstract then is ready to be photocopied and distributed to a selection committee. However, the same problems that prompted this effort are often encountered and points are deducted for qualitative research abstracts because there is an absence of a problem statement, of a hypothesis, and of statistics, as the format might call for.

Table 12-1 is offered as an alternative and provides for your encore. Table 12-2 offers a short exemplar of an actual qualitative research abstract, using the same study that has been used throughout the format book to demonstrate the research proposal and research report formats.

We would like to encourage you to submit an abstract of your research as soon as possible to as many of your discipline's conferences as you can. If you are a beginner researcher, these con-

Table 12-1   Outline for Qualitative Research Abstract

I—Aim of the Study	a) Phenomenon of interest.
	b) Relevance for discipline.
II—Evolution of the Study	a) Rational, experiential, and historical contents.
III—The Method of Inquiry: General	a) Brief overview of the purpose of the method.
	b) Basic steps.
	c) Suggestion for future inquiries.
IV—The Method of Inquiry: Applied	Brief overview of specific steps: sample, interviews, setting, procedures, consent, and data analysis.
V—Findings of the Study	Brief synopsis of the findings of the study.
VI—Reflection on the Findings	a) Brief synopsis of the meaning, understandings, and possible implications of the study.
	b) Significance and substance briefly discussed.

Table 12-2 Abbreviated Exemplar of Outline for Qualitative Research Abstract (Continuing With Anger Proposal)

I—Aim of the Study	a) Phenomenon. b) Relevance to nursing.	a) Understanding the meaning of anger. b) Without understanding grounded in the perceptions of those who have experienced anger and are willing to describe the various out comes, we do not have a basis for intervention for practice.
II—Evolution of the Study	a) Rationale, experiential, and historical contexts.	a) One might say that from the beginning of time anger has had its destructive force on both individuals and societies in politics and the personal domain of living.
III—The Method of Inquiry: General	a) Purpose and steps of the method.	a) Summarize the intent of this method, to understand the meaning of experience, where theory development concerning human beings must begin.
IV—The Method of Inquiry: Applied	a) Specific steps	a) Again summarize the interesting paths on which you were led and the variety of material used to facilitate a full understanding of your study, in this case anger. (See Table 9-2 for this study.)

Table 12-2 *(continued)*

V—Findings of the Study	Brief synopsis of the findings.	a) Anger makes people sick, especially if it is repressed. b) Anger that is repressed can be transformed into physiological, psychological, and/or social pathology or a combination. c) Anger is encouraged by society to be concealed. d) Some transformative manifestations of anger include obesity, gastrointestinal problems, headaches, hypertension, drug abuse, cardiac disease, anxiety, depression, self-destructive social patterns, low self-esteem, self-hatred, and domestic violence/other violence. e) Transformative conditions are treated with parallel treatments and the symptoms temporarily cured only to reoccur because the root problem was not addressed. Rarely does a transformative condition exist in isolation.
VI—Reflections on the Findings	Synopsis of meanings, significance, and implications.	"If anger goes unrecognized, it is left in silence. Repressed into recesses of the unconscious, it reappears transformed into something society finds more acceptable. Then society is spared the 'fury' of a woman and the condition can be treated. Even child abuse, it seems, is something less frightening than a woman's rage. We fail to see that child abuse is a woman's rage, that migraine headaches are an expression of anger, and that fury, as in furious, is at the heart of destructive relationships." Munhall (1994)

ferences offer you rich experiences of sharing your work, hearing other's work and developing a collegial network. Also, if you are a beginner please have others read your abstracts and think seriously about their suggestions.

If your research subject lends itself to it, we encourage you to offer to present your research to public policy groups or health interests groups and to the lay public. Look up community organizations where your subject might fit and give them a call. Most organizations welcome speakers and the often perceived separation of "town and gown" is held up to question, as researchers from universities gladly give talks to community groups.

We must hasten to warn you that just as a publication does, a selection committee has the distinct possibility of rejecting an abstract. Please do not let this discourage you. The first day is the hardest; you might experience an ego headache, but get up, dust off your boots (or is it knees?), and keep submitting. Often, conferences are overwhelmed with submissions, so make your abstract stand out. Reach out to others who present regularly for help with this. You will find faculty members who can assist you with this. The authors have both experienced the down one feels when an abstract or publication is rejected. I doubt that there is one faculty member who has not! Hope for an acceptance, if not the first time, the next time, or even the next time.

When you get your first acceptance for presentation or publication, your coaches here say, "Congratulations!"

In Closing

Using methods of qualitative research, the overall goal is to achieve accurate portrayal, authentic descriptions that enable understanding, and valid representation of the experience or cultures that you are studying. An important consideration, especially in regard to the scientific adequacy of the study, is to remain as close as feasible to the philosophical underpinnings and aims of the method. That is why a distinctive format in the proposal and report needs to be utilized in order to enhance the substance of the study, rather than manipulate the substance of the study to fit into a different form.

Placing qualitative research into quantitative research proposals is like trying to hammer a round peg idea into a square hole method. Researchers who use qualitative methods find themselves judged poorly because their study cannot be communicated clearly within the traditional, quantitative research format. Herein are suggested formats to encourage substance. And substance should be what research is all about in the first place.

Remember substance has to do with an *important aim*, *excellent* application of the method, deliberate and thoughtful reflection on your findings, accentuating the significance of your study, and a meaningful critique. Remember also the importance of original sources and immersing yourself in learning the philosophical underpinnings of your method, remember the sticky notes with your aim, remember to find the right faculty advisor and committee, and remember your English teacher and transitional sentences. Remember, too, to make sure you disseminate your research findings broadly and widely.

You might not believe it at this moment (perhaps some of you do) but the life of doing research, while not easy (and who wants easy anyway?) is intensely fascinating; it is a place to transcend yourself, to grow and to inspire. Research is challenging, and the first research project, such as a dissertation, is probably the most difficult one, but you will be gaining all sorts of stimulating practical and intellectual new insights. You will find meaning where meaning did not exist before. This adventure is worth it in every way, for what it gives to you and for what you ultimately give to others. When you complete your dissertation, you will not only have gained significant knowledge about the focus of your inquiry, you will have also gained important insight into yourself and your abilities. Nothing builds confidence like success. When you overcome the challenges you meet along the way in your dissertation journey, your confidence will grow, and somehow the journey will become less arduous! We congratulate you in anticipation of your impending success and wish you well on this journey.

And now, we send to you faith, hope, and confidence. We have faith, hope, and confidence that through your qualitative research, you will raise the consciousness of individuals and groups, you will help us understand that at the core of all things is meaning, and you will contribute to the liberation from oppression by questioning stereotypes, assumptions, and presuppositions. You will also find solutions to problems by listening to the voices and stories of those we serve, and you will discover the multitude of practices and policies that no longer work (if they ever did), and you will discover from the ground up new ones and means to a better quality of life for all. These are all tasks of no small consequence.

Qualitative Research Resources on the Web

Comprehensive Qualitative Research Sites

International Institute for Qualitative Methodology
http://www.uofaweb.ualberta.ca/iiqm/

International Institute of Human Understanding
http://www.iihu.org/

Intute: Research Tools and Methods
http://www.intute.ac.uk/socialsciences/research-tools/

Kerlins.net Qualitative Research page
http://kerlins.net/bobbi/research/qualresearch/

My Qualitative TiddlyWiki: A Reusable Non-Linear
Personal Web Notebook about All Things
Qualitative
http://technology-escapades.net/qualitative.htm

QualPage: Resources for Qualitative Research
http://www.qualitativeresearch.uga.edu/QualPage/

Qualitative Research in Information Systems
http://www.qual.auckland.ac.nz/

Specialized Qualitative Research Sites

Action Research Resources
http://www.scu.edu.au/schools/gcm/ar/arhome.html

AROW: Action and Research Open Web
http://www2.fhs.usyd.edu.au/arow/

Bridges: Mixed Methods Network for Behavioral, Social, and
Health Research
http://www.fiu.edu/~bridges/

Cochrane Qualitative Research Methods Group
http://www.joannabriggs.edu.au/cqrmg/index.html

Collaborative Action Research Network
http://www.did.stu.mmu.ac.uk/carn/

Computer Assisted Qualitative Data Analysis (CAQDAS)
Networking Project page
http://caqdas.soc.surrey.ac.uk/

Ethno/CA News: Information on Ethnomethodology and Conversation
Analysis
http://www.paultenhave.nl/EMCA.htm

Grounded Theory Institute
http://www.groundedtheory.org/

International Institute for Human Understanding
http://www.iihu.org

Narrative Psychology Internet and Resource Guide
http://web.lemoyne.edu/~hevern/narpsych.html

Online QDA
http://onlineqda.hud.ac.uk/index.php

Phenomenology Online
http://www.phenomenologyonline.com/

SSSI: Society for the Study of Symbolic Interaction
http://www.espach.salford.ac.uk/sssi/index.html

Online Discussion Groups

Qual-software
http://caqdas.soc.surrey.ac.uk/qualsoftware.htm

University of Georgia's Qualitative Interest Group (QUIG)
http://www.coe.uga.edu/quig/list.html

Online Journals

Forum: Qualitative Social Research (*FQS*)
http://www.qualitative-research.net/fqs/fqs-eng.htm

DAOL: Discourse Analysis Online
http://extra.shu.ac.uk/daol/index.html

The International Journal of Qualitative Methods
http://www.ualberta.ca/~ijqm/

The Qualitative Report (*TQR*)
http://www.nova.edu/ssss/QR/index.html

Social Research Update
http://www.soc.surrey.ac.uk/sru/

References

Anfara, V. A., Jr., Brown, K. M., & Mangione, T. L. (2002). Qualitative analysis on stage: Making the research process more public. *Educational Researcher, 31*(7), 28–38.

Atkinson, P. (1992). *Understanding ethnographic texts.* Newbury Park, CA: Sage.

Beebe, J. (2001). *Rapid assessment process: An introduction.* Walnut Creek, CA: AltaMira.

Bohm, D. (1985). *Unfolding meaning: A weekend of dialogue.* London: Routledge.

Chamberlain, J. (1999). Unpublished? Try your dissertation. *APA Monitor Online, 30*(11). Retrieved April 15, 2007, from http://apa.org/monitor/dec99/ed1.html

Cheek, J. (2002). Advancing what? Qualitative research, scholarship and the research imperative. *Qualitative Health Research, 12*(8), 1130–1140.

Chenail, R. J. (1995). Presenting qualitative data. *The Qualitative Report, 2*(3). Retrieved April 9, 2007, from http://www.nova.edu/ssss/QR/QR2-3/presenting.html

Chenail, R. J. (1997). Keeping things plumb in qualitative research. *The Qualitative Report, 3*(3). Retrieved April 9, 2007, from http://www.nova.edu/ssss/QR/QR3-3/plumb.html

Chenail, R. J. (2000). Navigating the "seven c's": Curiosity, confirmation, comparison, changing, collaborating, critiquing, and combinations. *The Qualitative Report, 4*(3/4). Retrieved April 9, 2007, from http://www.nova.edu/ssss/QR/QR4-3/sevencs.html

Chenail, R. (2005). Future directions for qualitative methods. In D. H. Sprenkle & F. Piercy (Eds.), *Research methods in family therapy* (2nd ed., pp. 191–208). New York: Guilford.

Chenail, R. J., & Maione, P. (1997). Sensemaking in clinical qualitative research. *The Qualitative Report, 3*(1). Retrieved April 9, 2007, from http://www.nova.edu/ssss/QR/QR3-1/sense.html

Clandinin, D. J. (Ed.). (2006). *Handbook of narrative inquiry: Mapping a methodology.* Thousand Oaks, CA: Sage.

Crang, M. A., & Cook, I. (2007). *Doing ethnographies.* London: Sage.

Creswell, J. W. (2002). *Educational research: Planning, conducting, and evaluating quantitative and qualitative research.* Upper Saddle River, NJ: Merrill Prentice Hall.

Creswell, J. (2003). *Research design: Qualitative, quantitative, and mixed methods approaches.* Thousand Oaks, CA: Sage.

Creswell, J. (2006). *Qualitative inquiry and research design: Choosing among five approaches* (2nd ed.). Thousand Oaks, CA: Sage Publications.

Critical Appraisal Skills Programme. (2002). *Making sense of evidence: 10 questions to help you make sense of qualitative research.* London: Milton Keynes Primary Trust Care. Retrieved September 17, 2007, from http://www.phru.uk/Doc_links/Qualitative%20Appraisal%20Tool.pdf

Crotty, M. (1998). *The foundations of social research: Meaning and perspective in the research process.* London: Sage.

Davies, D., & Dodd, J. (2002). Qualitative research and the question of rigor. *Qualitative Health Research, 12*(2), 279–289.

Dreyfus, H. (1972). *What computers can't do: A critique of artificial reason.* New York: Harper Row.

Drisko, J. W. (1997). Strengthening qualitative studies and reports: Standards to promote academic integrity. *Journal of Social Work Education, 33*(1), 185–198.

Ellis, C. (2004). *The ethnographic I: A methodological novel about autoethnography.* Walnut Creek, CA: AltaMira.

Georgi, A. (1970). *Psychology as a human science. A phenomenologically based approach.* New York: Harper & Row.

Germano, W. (2005). *From dissertation to book.* Chicago: University of Chicago Press.

Gilbert, K. R. (Ed.). (2000). *The emotional nature of qualitative research.* Boca Raton, FL: CRC Press.

Goulding, C. (2002). *Grounded theory: A practical guide for management, business and market researchers.* London: Sage.

Harry, B., Sturges, K. M., & Klingner, J. K. (2005). Mapping the process: An exemplar of process and challenge in grounded theory analysis. *Educational Researcher, 34*(2), 3–13.

Heath, H., & Cowley, S. (2004). Developing a grounded theory approach: A comparison of Glaser and Strauss. *International Journal of Nursing Studies, 41*(2), 141–150.

Herr, K. G., & Anderson, G. L. (2005). *The action research dissertation: A guide for students and faculty.* Thousand Oaks, CA: Sage.

Hutchison, S. (1993). The grounded theory method. In P. Munhall & C. B. Oiler (Eds.), *Nursing research: A qualitative perspective, 2nd Edition.* New York: National League of Nursing.

Kirk, J., & Miller, M. L. (1986). *Reliability and validity in qualitative research.* Beverly Hills, CA: Sage.

Laudan, L. (1977). *Progress and its Problems: Toward a theory of scientific growth.* Berkeley: University of California Press.

Lincoln, Y., & Guba, E. (1985). *Naturalistic inquiry.* Beverly Hills, CA: Sage.

Lincoln, Y. S., & Tierney, W. G. (2004). Qualitative research and institutional review boards. *Qualitative Inquiry, 10*(2), 219–234.

Lock, L. F., Silverman, S. J., & Spirduso, W. W. (2004). *Reading and understanding research* (2nd ed.). Thousand Oaks, CA: Sage.

Luey, B. (Ed.). (2004). *Revising your dissertation: Advice from leading editors.* Berkeley: The University of California Press.

Mackey, M. (2007). Evaluation of qualitative research. In P. L. Munhall (Ed.), *Nursing research: A qualitative perspective* (4th ed., pp. 555–568). Sudbury, MA: Jones and Bartlett.

Mahrer, A. R., & Boulet, D. B. (1999). How to do discovery-oriented psychotherapy research. *Journal of Clinical Psychology, 55*(12), 1481–1493.

Marshall, C., & Rossman, G. B. (2006). *Designing qualitative research* (4th ed.). Thousand Oaks, CA: Sage Publications.

Mays, N., & Pope, C. (2000). Assessing quality in qualitative research. *BMJ, 320,* 50–52.

McNiff, J., & Whitehead, J. (2002). *Action research: Principles and practice* (2nd ed.). London: RoutledgeFalmer.

Merleau-Ponty, M. (1956). What is phenomenology? *Cross Currents, 6,* 59–70.

Morse, J. M. (2002). Enhancing the usefulness of qualitative inquiry: Gaps, direction, and responsibilities. *Qualitative Health Research, 12*(10), 1419–1426.

Munhall, P. (1988). Ethical considerations in qualitative research. *Western Journal of Nursing Research, 10*(2), 150–162.

Munhall, P. (1993). Women's anger and its meanings: A phenomenological perspective. *Health Care for Women International, 14*(6), 481–491.

Munhall, P. (1994a). *Revisioning phenomenology: Nursing and health science research.* Sudbury, MA: Jones and Bartlett.

Munhall, P. (1994b). The transformation of anger into pathology. In P. Munhall (Ed.), *In Women's Experience.* New York: National League for Nursing Press.

Munhall, P. (1995). Anger in women. In P. Munhall (Ed.), *In Women's Experience.* (Vol. 1). Sudbury, MA: Jones and Bartlett Publishers.

Munhall, P. (1998). Qualitative designs. In P. Brink & M. Wood (Eds.), *Advanced designs in nursing research* (2nd ed.). Newbury Park, CA: Sage.

Munhall, P. (2000). Unknowing. In W. Kelly & V. Fitzsimons (Eds.), *Understanding cultural diversity.* Sudbury, MA: Jones and Bartlett.

Munhall, P. (2002). Transformation of anger by men. In P. Munhall & Madden (Eds.), *The Emergence of Man into the 21st Century.* Sudbury, MA: Jones and Bartlett.

Munhall, P. (2007a). *Nursing research: A qualitative perspective* (4th ed.). Sudbury, MA: Jones and Bartlett.

Munhall, P. (2007b). A phenomenological method. In P. Munhall (Ed.), *Nursing Research: A qualitative perspective* (4th ed., pp. 145–210). Sudbury, MA: Jones and Bartlett.

National Research Council. (2002). *Scientific research in education.* Washington, DC: National Academy Press.

Omery, A. (1983). Phenomenology: A method for nursing research. *Advances in Nursing Science, 5*(2), 49–63.

Patton, M. Q. (1990). *Qualitative evaluation and research methods* (2nd ed.). Newbury Park, CA: Sage.

Russell, C. K., & Gregory, D. M. (2003). Evaluation of qualitative research studies. *Evidence-Based Nursing, 6*(2), 36–40.

Ryan, G. W., & Bernard, H. R. (2003). Techniques to identify themes. *Field Methods, 15*(1), 85–109.

Sanday, P. (1983). The ethnographic paradigm. In M. van Manen (Ed.), *Qualitative methodology* (pp. 19–36). Beverly Hills, CA: Sage Publications.

Sandelowski, H. (1986). The problem of rigor in qualitative research. *Advances in Nursing Science, 8*(3), 27–31.

Schutz, A. (1970). In H. Wagner (Ed.), *On phenomenology and social relations.* Chicago: University of Chicago Press.

Schwandt, T. A. (2007). *The Sage dictionary of qualitative inquiry* (3rd ed.). Thousand Oaks, CA: Sage.

Seale, C. (1999). *The quality of qualitative research.* London: Sage.

Speigelberg, H. (1976). *The phenomenological movement, Vol. I & II.* The Hague, Netherlands: Martinus Nijhoff.

Strauss, A. L., & Corbin, J. M. (1998). *Basics of qualitative research: Techniques and procedures for developing grounded theory* (2nd ed.). Thousand Oaks, CA: Sage.

Stringer, E. T. (2007). *Action research* (3rd ed.). Thousand Oaks, CA: Sage.

Tang, Y., & Joiner, C. (Eds.). (2006). *Synergic inquiry: A collaborative action methodology*. Thousand Oaks, CA: Sage.

Van Kaam, A. (1969). *Existential foundation of psychology*. New York: Doubleday.

van Manen, M. (1984). Practicing phenomenological writing. *Phenomenology and Pedagogy, 2*(1), 36–69.

van Manen, M. (1990). *Researching the lived experience*. Buffalo: State University of New York Press.

van Manen, M. (2002). *Writing in the dark. Phenomenological studies in interpretive inquiry*. Ontario, Canada: Althouse Press.

Whittemore, R., Chase, S. K., & Mandle, C. L. (2001). Validity in qualitative research. *Qualitative Health Research, 11*(4), 522–537.

Wolcott, H. F. (1994). *Transforming qualitative data: Description, analysis, and interpretation*. Thousand Oaks, CA: Sage.

Yin, R. K. (2003). *Case study research* (3rd ed.). Thousand Oaks, CA: Sage.

Dissertation Proposals

PERSPECTIVES OF ETHICAL CARE:
A GROUNDED THEORY APPROACH

by
Patricia Hentz Becker

Dissertation Committee:

Professor Patricia Munhall, Sponsor
Approved by the Committee on the Degree of
Doctor of Education
Date: _____

Submitted in partial fulfillment of the requirements for the Degree of Doctor of Education in
Teachers College, Columbia University

TABLE OF CONTENTS

NURSES' PERCEPTIONS OF MAKING MISTAKES IN CLINICAL PRACTICE: A PHENOMENOLOGICAL PERSPECTIVE

by
Gretchen Almquist-Copeland

Dissertation Committee:

Professor Patricia Munhall, Sponsor
Approved by the Committee on the Degree of Doctor of Education
Date: _____

Submitted in partial fulfillment of the requirements for the Degree of Doctor of Education in Teachers College, Columbia University

TABLE OF CONTENTS

LIVING THROUGH THE DEATH OF A WISHED-FOR BABY: A PHENOMENOLOGICAL PERSPECTIVE TO UNDERSTANDING MOTHERS' EXPERIENCES FOLLOWING PERINATAL DEATH/LOSS

by
Sarah Steen Lauterbach

Dissertation Committee:

Professor Patricia Munhall, Sponsor
Professor Marilyn Rawnsley
Approved by the Committee on the Degree of Doctor of Education
Date: _____

Submitted in partial fulfillment for the requirements for the Degree of Doctor of Education in Teachers College, Columbia University

TABLE OF CONTENTS

Dissertation Outlines

PERSPECTIVES OF ETHICAL CARE: A GROUNDED THEORY APPROACH

by
Patricia Hentz Becker

Dissertation Committee:

Professor Patricia Munhall, Sponsor
Professor Herve Varenne
Approved by the Committee on the Degree of
Doctor of Education
Date: _____

Submitted in partial fulfillment of the requirements for the Degree of Doctor of Education in Teachers College, Columbia University

Table of Contents

NURSES' EXPERIENTIAL PERSPECTIVES OF MISTAKE MAKING IN CLINICAL PRACTICE

by Gretchen Almquist-Copeland

Dissertation Committee:

Professor Patricia Munhall, Sponsor
Professor Susan Salmond
Approved by the Committee on the Degree of Doctor of Education
Date: _____

Submitted in partial fulfillment of the requirements for the Degree of Doctor of Education in Teachers College, Columbia University

Table of Contents

IN ANOTHER WORLD: A PHENOMENOLOGICAL PERSPECTIVE AND DISCOVERY OF MEANING IN MOTHERS' EXPERIENCE OF DEATH OF A WISHED-FOR BABY

by
Sarah Steen Lauterbach

Dissertation Committee:

Professor Patricia Munhall, Sponsor
Professor Elizabeth Maloney
Approved by the Committee on the Doctor of Education
Date: _____

Submitted in partial fulfillment of the requirements for the Degree of Doctor of Education in Teachers College Columbia University

Table of Contents

Index